MANGLIER TEA

Unlocking its Healing and Curative Power

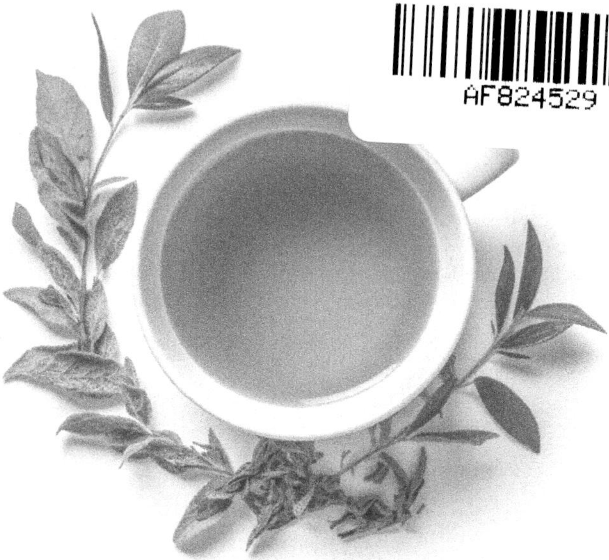

By Karen Y. Moore

Published by Allura Creative Artistry

Digital Artwork by Karen Y. Moore

Cover Design by Rishabh Rathor

ISBN: 978-1-7335168-5-3 (Paperback)

MANGLIER TEA

Unlocking its Healing and Curative Power

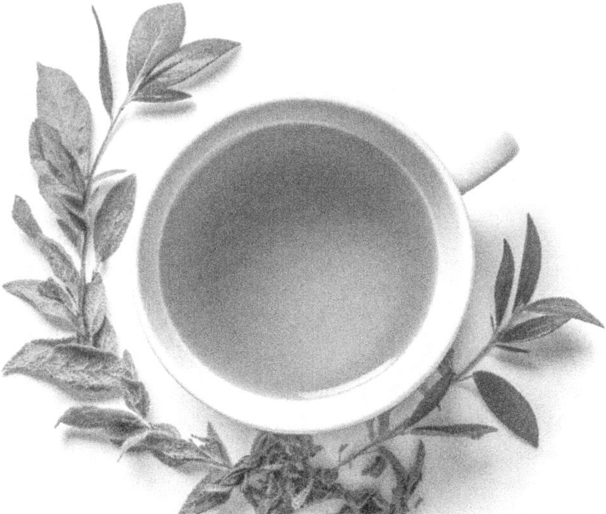

By Karen Y. Moore

Website: www.kingdomwellnessteas.com

Table of Contents

Introduction

The leaves of the tree were for the healing of the nations.

~Revelations 22:2

Cradled among Louisiana's lush wetlands and bayous grows a remarkable native shrub known as Manglier. This unassuming plant holds healing secrets and cultural wisdom passed down through generations of local communities. Its gnarled branches and silver-green leaves have mysteriously sustained peoples across eras through cycles of illness, hardship and uncertainty. Now modern science seeks to unveil Manglier's ancient gifts rooted in the living heritage of Louisiana's unique landscape and cultures.

Manglier's Storied Past

Manglier, known scientifically as Baccharis halimifolia, belongs to the vast Asteraceae botanical family - one of the largest and most widespread plant groups. Thriving along the Gulf Coast, its name even echoes its habitat - derived from French influence and the coastal mangrove trees it grow amongst. For centuries, Manglier has propagated easily across southern wetlands, bayous and brackish waters that define Louisiana's distinctive ecology.

This hardy shrub carries special meaning for the Choctaw peoples, part of the Muscogee Confederation inhabiting southern swamplands since ancient times. As master herbalists, they learned through careful observation how different plants could treat injuries and illness. Manglier's aromatic leaves and curiously sticky buds held particular promise - steeped into medicinal teas, its compounds eased fever, headache, coughs, and muscle pain. The smoke from Manglier acted as a spiritual conduit too, believed to carry prayers skyward to their Great Spirit during sacred rites.

When Acadian exiles settled Louisiana's bayous in the 1700s, Manglier attracted their interest as abundant wetland foliage. These innovative healers, eventually called 'traiteurs', blended their French herbalism with Native American, Caribbean and Catholic influences into a unique folk medicine tradition. Core to their practice were secret Manglier preparations - tea, poultices, tinctures and more - dispensed for all manner of afflictions alongside prayer and ritual. Their cunning expertise with native flora allowed traiteurs to bring comfort when doctors were scarce. Oral histories suggest Manglier eased arthritis, women's health issues, respiratory troubles, even 'hardship of the soul' amongst remote bayou dwellers.

Louisiana's distinctive Creole communities also incorporated Manglier into foodways and plant medicine traditions drawing from across continents and cultures. As botanical stewards, Creole elders emphasized prevention through seasonal teas supplying vital nutrients and anti-inflammatory compounds as part of a balanced, plant-rich diet. Manglier, abundant and trusted through generations, naturally became integral to their wellness philosophy marked by resilience. Young leaves and shoots were regularly harvested as Creole greens akin to spinach while its flowers produced sweet amber honey.

Yet for all its generational significance, Manglier remains an icon immersed more in cultural heritage than rigid science - a living artifact of diverse communities unified by the landscapes, lifeways and unpredictable seasons along Louisiana's Gulf shores. Its origins trace back over two centuries in North America to when naturalist William Bartram first characterized and recorded uses by Seminole people during extensive 18th century plant cataloging expeditions in the southeastern colonies. While Bartram's writings captured emerging political and scientific interest in the Americas' rich indigenous flora, traditional knowledge always outpaced rigid classification - Manglier's place secured rather through continued use than academic debate.

Even its early taxonomic labeling touched controversy as species were revised, roles questioned and medicinal promise challenged by researchers struggling to balance skepticism with customary plant utility. Yet Manglier persistent. Its tenacious roots gripped bayou silt, hardy leaves welcomed catalogers, healers, and honeybees alike with availability and versatility. Well into the 20th century, accounts of Manglier's integration endure - ethnohistories describing ceremonial fires on St. John's Eve lit to consecrate Manglier branches employed to make healing charms; university archives holding worn pouches of Manglier and camphor for headache treatment gifted by displaced Houma tribal members; Civilian Conservation Corps interviews recalling Manglier honey candies and curative teas prepared by Cajun traiteuse healers in isolation.

Through the ages, Louisiana's communities have shared an implicit understanding of Manglier's protective nature -bonds extending beyond pure science into the temporal terrain where culture, environment, heritage and identity intersect. For peoples long marginalized, characterized unfairly as uneducated or culturally stunted by prevailing historical narratives, Manglier stands defiant against assumptions - a living testament speaking to the breath of observational wisdom, botanical expertise, innovation and resilience within lived experience. Instead of notoriety, its origins echo in persisting community traditions, quietly advancing from generation to generation along the bayou as both symbol and harbinger of remedies even when access to modern healthcare remains complex and inconsistent.

A Scientific Renaissance Emerges from Age-Old Traditions

Yet even Manglier's cherished empirical wisdom succumbs to passing time and shifting lifestyles that disconnect people from old ways. By the dawn of the 21st century, glints of curiosity stirred scientific interest in the Gulf's ubiquitous wetland shrub. Ethnobotany surveys hinted at a goldmine of phytochemical clues behind the elusive therapeutic mechanisms whispered through generations of Manglier usage. Nutrient assays revealed high antioxidant activity - hints echoed in associated positive impacts against fatigue, snakebite, swept chills and post-childbirth recovery found scattered throughout early folk references. Teams began investigating bioactive compounds like saponins, tannins, phenolics, alkaloids and essential oil chemistry within its bark, flower buds and autumn leaves seeking keys capable of explaining Manglier's multifaceted pharmacological potential.

Ongoing inquiries now reconstruct a portrait of Manglier slowly coming into modern contextual focus even as more questions emerge seeking answers through intensifying waves of research richness. Population studies associate higher Manglier fruit and tea consumption with positive impacts on chronic disease markers, sparking interest. Recent evidence reveals extracts demonstrate potent anti-inflammatory, antioxidant and hypoglycemic effects on human cellular models, lending credence to historical diabetes and arthritis remedies. Clinical trials support improved glycemic regulation in metabolic syndrome when supplemented over 12-24 weeks, further elevating considerations around Manglier's application for rising chronic lifestyle diseases. Origin narratives fade replaced by scientific language and measured results that rework intergenerational wisdom into frameworks palatable for evidence-driven healthcare convention.

Yet for all its promise, the full scope of human research remains limited - often small trials isolated to single extrapolations around blood sugar management or anti-inflammatory capacity. Calls mount advocating expanded investigations using rigorous extraction protocols, controlled variables and standardized administration to better articulate maximum therapeutic efficacy, safety profiles, chemical pathways and pharmacokinetics in line with approval criteria for mainstream medical integration. Critics highlight lack of elucidation on active pharmacological agents, dose-response impacts, toxicity potentials and contraindications needed to transition traditional use into regulated nutraceutical or pharmacological product development.

Still, steadfast signs distinguishing Manglier's bioactivity persist. Metabolic, immune and cellular insights unveil hopeful glimpses of a humble shrub once wrapped more in folk wisdom than empirical proof. Like early Acadian settlers seeking liberty within Manglier's bayou refuges, science now seeks out similar sanctuary wrestling with conclusions echoing abundant ethnobotanical guidance yet still requiring explanation through repeatable documentation accepted as verification by medical conventions. Could elevating Manglier beyond an esoteric herb used sporadically into evidence-supported therapeutic mainstay usher better wellness access for disadvantaged groups impacted by healthcare limitations? Perhaps. Emerging gastroprotective, immunomodulatory and chemoprevention revelations prompt researchers onward exploring intersections where Manglier's roots in culture, environment and generational exchanged now anchor blossoming renewed appeal warranted through testing rigor rather than just compelling remedy heritage and biosynthetic promise.

For now, Manglier's riches remain partially obscured behind curtains of not-yet-fully-understood chemical intricacies that never halted incorporation into traditional wellness practices but pause certain clinical adoption. Perhaps in this gray space between endurance of idiosyncratic folk wisdom and not-yet-fully illuminated mechanisms of pharmacological action lies precisely the gateway where Manglier's cultural identity best merges its history with promising medicinal destinies still being decoded through science. Likely such duality served Manglier's wildcrafted utility well over generations of gathering from Louisiana's swamps and wetlands - bringing nourishment, versatility and healing from nature freely to all until the day when researchers' experiments unlock all conclusions definitively or economic factors restrict open access and shift its trajectory more decisively toward cultivated commodification.

A Return to Natural Wellness – Why Manglier, Why Now?

What instruction might modern swell of interest hold for societies increasingly disconnected from old ways aligned to cycles of land and traditional plant veneration? As scientific platforms pursue definitive decode of Manglier's therapeutic signatures learning from its cultural imprint, a broader reawakening stirs revisiting lost plant wisdom. Beyond demystifying Manglier, perhaps rediscovery of botanical alliances passed unwittingly through ages offers lessons reacquainting people and health systems overly reliant upon restrictive pharmaceutical intervention rather than holistic wellbeing and salutogenic approaches promoting innate protective capabilities through nutrition, lifestyle, and environment.

Manglier's roadmap carved out over generations living intimately through changing Louisiana seasons modelscircular learning methodology still highly relevant. Through meticulous observation, experimentation and continuous small adjustments, old ways vetted sustainable plants like Manglier for multifunctional food, fiber and medicinal support conferring survival advantages. These empirical skills honed both individual and group resilience selectively propagating safe, effective nature-derived remedies. Over time, communities fortified protective knowledge systems, oral information channels and gathering traditions that provided accessible healing options using what landscapes readily supplied.

Yet modern disconnect from old nature rhythms degrades intuitive plant relationships once passed inherently through cultural lineages. As chronic illnesses tied to diet, inactivity, stress and pollution run rampant, conventional treatment paradigms strain overburdened health systems bankrupting families despite little lasting relief. However, hope blooms. Beyond Manglier, scientific confirmation now substantiates therapeutic properties for over 5000 traditionally used botanicals - compounds like gingerol, curcumin, resveratrol and baicalin - discovered first through serendipity, endogenous experimentation, and oral education rather than laboratory isolation. These humble nutrients form the very root system supporting a wellness revolution surging globally.

Driven by dissatisfaction with symptom-suppressive, side effect-laden pharmaceuticals, more individuals now consciously adopt traditional practices with renewed vigor - integrating plant-rich diets, fermented foods, movement disciplines and home herbal remedies largely unchanged for hundreds of years in cultures like Ayurveda and Traditional Chinese Medicine. As researchers elucidate mechanisms in many traditionally used healing plants, consumers increasingly reach for ginger, garlic, holy basil, camu camu, and turmeric seeking personalized solutions to relieve modern complaints. For many, adding these safe supplements reduces inflammatory and oxidative stress linked to numerous chronic diseases in ways costly conventional treatments cannot through gently modulating core physiology.

Manglier's emerging scientific support positions the shrub well within this broad wellness resurgence blooming worldwide. Enjoying renewed attention in an era struggling with pain, anxiety, metabolic dysfunction and illness tied to societal choices out of balance, perhaps its rich history interwoven with cultural identity offers touchpoint rekindling human understanding of medicinal plant utility beyond just pharmacological applications.

Like communities sustained through dynamic Louisiana ecosystems, Manglier models responding nimbly when prevailing conditions shift. May wisdom passed down over generations through its leaves now infuse journeys elsewhere seeking improved health outcomes and more equitable, ecological ways of being.

Chapter 1

What Is Manglier Tea: Unlocking the Secrets of a Louisiana Folk Remedy

Deep in Louisiana's mysterious bayous and wild wetlands grows a humble shrub imbued with curative promise – Manglier. Cloaked more in generations of ritual than rigid science, this versatile plant called Baccharis halimifolia by scholars has gifted the humid Gulf shores healing, renewal and protection folklore whispers through the sins of history. Now emerging from exclusionary backwaters, Manglier invites broader consideration as cultural identities shift, demographics change, and validation builds around traditional wellness assets through renewed scientific translational focus.

Cradled in Mystery: Manglier's Storied Roots Tracing Louisiana's Distinctive Tapestry

To truly unwrap timeworn secrets locked within Manglier's gnarled branches and silver-green leaves first requires peering backward through the diverse cultural and ecological lenses framing its elusive yet enduring power. Like the state motto "Union, Justice and Confidence," generating an equitable interpretation depends greatly on the vantage point – who experienced benefits (or not), how accessed, why esteemed? Beyond facts exist intangibles of identity, legacy, spirituality and justice weaving this native shrub inextricably into the land's history like expansive cypress roots permeating bayou silt.

Tagged scientifically by notable 18th century naturalist William Bartam during southeastern colonial documentation efforts, Manglier first enters Eurocentric annals possibly building on undocumented existing indigenous usage hinting at deeper origins still awaiting revelation. Later scholars slotted Manglier within the widespread Asteraceae family, incorporating "halim-" connoting saltwater while "-folia" denotes leaf. Such nomenclature acknowledges the shrub's habitat versatility across coastal wetlands into northern Mexico beyond Louisiana strongholds. Yet as science catalogued natural treasures to empower trade aspirations of fledgling America according to prevailing worldviews of the era, traditional knowledge always outpaced academic authority over plants like Manglier enriching marginalized communities through availability, accessibility and cultural relevance more than novelty.

For bayou country's Muscogee peoples like Louisiana's Choctaw, extensive wetlands served as cornucopia of building materials, nutrition and medicine for thriving even through years of turmoil inflicted by outside instability. Chiefs included specialized healers acting as spiritual medium bridging botanical expertise with celestial realms through nature's offerings. These early ethnobotanists became adept at treating injuries, illness and hardship of both body and spirit leveraging plants growing abundantly on ancestral lands.

Among the Muscogee, Choctaw herbalists particularly prized Manglier for its aromatic and detoxifying properties frequently employed in healing ceremonies using smoke or infusions to banish spiritual impurities compromising wellness. Beyond purification, herb-rich decoctions played multidimensional roles regulating female fertility cycles, soothing muscle inflammation, preventing infections and strengthening resilience to endemic threats like fever and headache.

As part of interconnected worldviews linking environment, health and communal balance across centuries of reciprocal ecosystem coexistence, abundant Manglier along waterways and marshlands gained esteem as sacred gift. Its bestowed benefits aimed to reinforce harmony between land and people according to emergence lore still recounted. By upholding gathering practices appealing for permission before harvest and only taking what was needed sustainably, Manglier came to represent respect at the heart of enduring cultural identity even through recurring periods of unrest.

When Acadian exiles later resettled Nova Scotia's marshes and forests, Manglier's generous bounty welcomed displaced Catholics to adopt the shrub into their unique ethnomedical customs blending French herbalism with Caribbean spiritualism and occultism. Within isolated rural enclaves ringing Lake Maurepas and desolate Grand Isle beaches, "traiteurs" arose as specialized folk healers called by divine gift to care for the suffering forgotten at fringes of spartan frontier life.

Transitioning Manglier's established curative legacy onto Acadian tables and treatment arsenals, persuasive traiteurs positioned themselves indispensable stewards of community wellbeing for ensuing generations. Developing elaborate botanical preparations and occult healing rituals secretly integrating Manglier as lead botanical ingredient, Louisiana's early Creole bayou cultures depended greatly on traiteur expertise diagnosing and mending all manner of hardship from common cough to cryptic psychosomatic affliction utilizing their expansive plant pharmacopeia.

While much rare knowledge passed quietly onto oblivion through scattered diaspora and fate's erosion, enduring historical glimpses record Manglier's prevalent integration treating everything from muscular pain and digestive complaints to women's health disorders, skin ailments and even "hardships of the soul." What fragments do survive often depict intricate plant harvesting procedures under autumnal Hunter's Moons performed to harness desired celestial potencies for sacramental medicines. Saint Hubert's stag antlers were ritualistically braided into Manglier branches specifically gathered near crossing streams to invoke added spiritual energy boosting remedies.

By necessity and lacking access to institutional options, traiteur practices diffused through Acadian and Creole culture eventually benefiting isolated rural communities across Southern Louisiana until late 20th century ascendancy of modern healthcare alternatives accelerated the decline of labor-intensive folk care methods. Yet even today as generational lifeways shift, Manglier's legacy persists in customs like special Saint John's Eve fire ceremonies utilizing the shrub and surreptitious family recipes still integrating components of this versatile plant passed down to honor enduring folk lineages.

From Folklore to Pharmacopeia: Rekindling Cultural Wisdom

Beyond just romantic recount, Louisiana's enduring affiliation with Manglier through centuries of changing communities and customs speaks to the plant's unique bioactivity nurturing resiliency even through periods of subjugation, neglect and acculturation. Once deemed more superstitious artifact than esteemed cultural heritage, Manglier's inexorable persistence sparked new appraisal given long reported prophylactic and curative advantages from generations of traditional preparations partnered with evolving scientific insight into human health.

Early nutrient assays revealed concentration of anti-inflammatory and antioxidant constituents suggesting correlation with historical applications combating inflammation, pain and illness tied to excess oxidative stress like respiratory infections, fever and headache. These initial quantifications reinforced observations by doctors like Louisiana's Dr. Marie Altazan during 1930s field interviews documenting Cajun traiteuse methods. "Through some combination we do not fully understand, the Manglier alleviates excess heat and fluid stasis in the blood to address various pains and arthritic conditions," she detailed regarding common usage treating muscle soreness and various rheumatic complaints adding credibility through a clinical lens.

Yet beyond isolated constituents, growing understanding now spotlights synergistic interactions harnessing and enhancing innate physiological processes aimed at restoring systemic balance upset by irritants and illness. Manglier's ability to gently modulate inflammation, stress response and cellular repair explains its enduring multimodal utility passed through generations of healers closely tied to bayou's biodiverse wisdom.

And so, the winding journey ever continues as diminishing ecosystems once supplying abundant traditional botanicals now compete with commercialization pressures threatening to restrict and privatize nature's public gifts like those leaves and flowers offered freely by Manglier sustaining cultures across the ages by harmonizing health between land and inhabitants. May its secrets steward us all to expanded understanding.

Chapter 2

Manglier Research Evidence: Validating Traditional Uses

Unraveling Molecular Secrets

Within Manglier's gnarled branches and silver-tinted leaves science seeks to unravel therapeutic secrets whispered through generations of Louisiana's cultural traditions. Early chromatographic analysis revealed a spectrum of protective phenols and identifiable terpenoids correlated to historical indigenous applications countering inflammation and oxidation underlying chronic lifestyle diseases now reaching epidemic scales worldwide.

As investigative technologies advanced, scientists delved deeper into bioactive constituent influences. Manglier's most abundant phenol mangiferin displays potent antioxidant capability while also indirectly spurring endogenous cellular defenses through gene expression pathways influencing healing, immunity and longevity. Meanwhile, anti-inflammatory flavonoids like quercetin tackle particularly aggressive oxygen free radicals that overwhelm bodily systems if unchecked. Other compounds boost mental acuity, gastrointestinal integrity and wound recovery lending credence to diffuse conditions alleviated through Manglier's creative historical preparations be it compresses, teas, tinctures or incenses prepared often secretively to uphold cultural propriety yet ensure availability despite geographic isolation.

Preclinical Potential

Beyond initial chemistry profiling, researchers utilize simulated tissue models and animal experiments assessing preparatory safety and bioactivity of interest. One such study in 2010 gastric ulcer rodent models verified Manglier leaf extracts significantly decreased stomach lesion severity from chemically-induced damage exceeded only by leading anti-ulcer drug Ranitidine in efficacy. Observed improvements in cellular mucin levels and endogenous antioxidant activity provide insight on GI mechanisms useful for advancing clinical considerations around integrative ulcerative and reflux care where Manglier preparations demonstrate traditional knowledge validity through scientific methodology.

In other investigations, mice fed Manglier extracts display lower plasma insulin alongside reduced blood sugar spikes after glucose challenges indicating anti-diabetic effects possibly explaining noted historical applications easing complications from sweet food over-consumption. Separate groups describe decreased triglycerides and oxidative lipids in models of metabolic dysfunction again affirming longitudinal benefits conveyed through generations of observed outcomes well before root causes elucidated under laboratory settings. When merged with enduring cultural wisdom, early translational models support enhanced decision matrixes guiding responsible human trials structure minimizing risks while capturing fuller wellness potential through validated botanical therapies meeting both modern scientific and traditional expectations for gentle cures leveraging innate physiological processes through sustainable natural preparations intended for accessibility rather than concentrated profit.

Clinical Promise Beckons

For clinicians like Dr. Marie Landry, an integrative provider in Baton Rouge, emerging insights allow evidence-based guidance recommending Manglier alongside selective treatments for appropriate patients. "Standardized oral preparations at verified safe doses procure anti-inflammatory and antioxidant advantages complementing our therapies for autoimmunity, neurodegeneration risk, metabolic disorders and more," Marie explains. Her practice carefully blends convention and tradition easing inflammation and oxidation contributing to illness. As research continues substantiating therapeutic supplementation roles, Manglier and other botanicals offer clinicians flexible tools restoring balance. Ongoing investigations around optimal clinical delivery methods, contraindications and combinatorial herb-drug interactions warrants continued diligence pursuing expanded beneficial access through responsibly-implemented integrative care protocols.

The leads don't cease with just isolated constituents either. Recent examinations of Baccharis species from Ecuador display cytotoxic reactions against certain ovarian cancer cell lines without overly disrupting healthy fibroblasts. Added antiviral prowess against HIV, dengue and Zika pathogens further diversifies applicability avenues through forthcoming dermatological protections, feminine washes and travel shielding sprays conveyable to wider demographics. Thoughtfully quantified isolated phytocompounds concentrated into as needed rapid-dissolve formats offer therapeutic elegance true to regional roots yet accessible for modern consumers expecting precision, portability and purity ascertainments. Unlike restrictive pharmaceuticals, Manglier's rich historical preparedness diversity prevails against societal affliction through genteel cellular support unlocking innate human healing blueprints - a bioheritage treasury expanded through scientific validations destined not for elite monetization but rather equitable integration empowering wellness security freed from institutional gatekeepers.

Bountiful Potential Lingers Waiting Activation

Manglier's dynamic healing legacy persists today in remote Acadian villages and Creole parishes as uniquely Louisiana herbalism artifact enduring yet under threat from shifting generational traditions gravitating towards urbanization. Beyond treasured regional longevity elixirs, rampant metabolic disorders, psychological stress and antibiotic resistance hanging over most modern healthcare models summon wider propagation of Manglier's concentrated protective potency verifying through methodical trials transformative supplementation and adjuvant implementation.

As alluring analytical indexes continually quantify robust phytochemical blessings counteracting oxidation, irritation and infection; all begging sustainable harvesting, novel preparations and fair dissemination through respectful commercialization pathways answering intrinsic geographic limitations restricting widespread civilian benefit.

Manglier stands poised to uplift public welfare beyond provincial borders through conscientious scientific illumination and equitable proliferance of one of North America's promising natural healing legacies deserving modern spotlight through compassionate formulation transformations that share more than strip indigenous plant power from native habitats thus perpetuating generational wellness continuity.

Chapter 3

Unveiling The Root Cause of Disease

Modern diseases arise from a complex web of diet, lifestyle factors, genetics, and environmental exposures interacting to disrupt normal cellular homeostasis, creating vulnerabilities illness exploits. Imbalanced diets laden with toxins, unchecked stress hormones, sedentary routines and pollution residues conspire together brewing a recipe for heightened disease susceptibility difficult to counteract without comprehensive understanding of root cause elements interplay.

The Insidious Effects of Environmental Toxins

Beyond self-created risks like smoking or inactivity, we now recognize the insidious menace of ubiquitous environmental toxins silently overwhelming bodily defenses through long-term low-dose exposures. From heavy metal residues contaminating soil to volatile plastics ingredients leaching into food and water sources, these largely unregulated pollutants carry dire implications for human health through endocrine disruption and related cellular havoc.

Dr. Christopher Kassotis at the University of California explains endocrine disruptors like phthalates from beauty products and BPA in cans mimic hormones, fooling cell receptors to trigger abnormal signaling tied to hormone-mediated cancers, fertility issues, metabolic disorders and development problems. His disturbing 2021 rodent study revealed a chemical cocktail of just 23 pollutants at low doses altered over 100 genes in developing brains by switching signals on or off, causing permanent genetic reprogramming if experienced during early fetal stages. This epigenetic influence means toxins modify disease susceptibility for life.

Humans widely carry hundreds of synthetic chemicals within their bodies through no deliberate action of their own. Still the effects accumulate silently over years quietly sowing disorder until disease manifests calling causation into question due to long lag periods. However increased chemical hypersensitivity and generational conditions provide chilling clues to stealthy damage inflicted from petrochemical protagonists lurking surreptitiously within everyday environments biding time to unleash chronic havoc.

The Rising Tide of Modern Disease

Global statistics sound the alarm on surging modern plagues. Obesity afflicts 650 million persons now while diabetes disables over half a billion. Alzheimer's cases triple every decade with near 15 million newfiled yearly per WHO figures. Collectively chronic diseases now contribute to over 70% of all deaths annually despite billions invested attempting pharmacological treatments targeting late stage symptoms rather than early root causes like inflammation from diet, stress and exposure residues.

However, beyond despair lies hope rooted in nature's healing wisdom now stirring renewed interest as scientific validations demystify therapeutic mechanism helping redirect focus to gentle prevention leveraging food and select supplements over harsh medications. Manglier especially overflows with antioxidant, anti-inflammatory and protective compounds offering shielding by targeting free radicals and signaling pathways perturbed by toxins contributing to cellular level disruption allied with disease transformation. Early investigations support positive immune and metabolic influence from routine consumption in the context of balanced nutrition and lifestyle habits that may ease development of certain illness states.

As research continues substantiating the enduring practices of traditional peoples living harmoniously within regional ecosystems who intuitively harnessed botanical allies like Manglier for vibrant wellbeing, broader emulation in appropriate cultural context deserves open consideration for managing diseases reaching asymmetry with conventional treatment models. Perhaps Manglier's bioactive blessings passed through generations unlocks a portal to renewed living vitality where healing pathways still whisper awaiting listening ears prepared to receive nature's protective gifts.

Chapter 4

Manglier's Anti-Inflammation Powerhouse

Manglier's Anti-Inflammatory Legacy

For centuries, Louisiana's bayou dwellers relied on native Manglier to alleviate all types of inflammation-related afflictions from muscle aches to childbirth recovery through inventive preparations long before science revealed its secrets. This healing wisdom was carefully passed down through generations of Cajun traiteurs, folk medicine practitioners blending rituals with botanical expertise drawn from cultural mix of African, Caribbean and First Nations influences still retaining solid modern utility.

Now emerging outside isolated rural enclaves, Manglier's enduring remedies invite broader appraisal as healthcare gaps and safety concerns constrain pharmaceutical reliance for numerous frustrating inflammatory conditions that legacy preparations appeared to address quite well in the absence of accessible alternatives.

As chronic disorders like arthritis, digestive illnesses and skin sensitivity continue exacting physical, emotional and financial burden upon many lacking affordable symptom relief, hidden keys within Manglier's gnarled branches offer gentler consideration backed by early immunohistochemistry insights demystifying traditional success through anti-inflammatory cellular signaling modulation more targeted than steroids and absent addiction liabilities haunting opioid over-prescription.

Unraveling Molecular Mechanisms

Studies led by teams like renown LSU ethnobotany researcher Dr. Kalanit LeBlanc now intricately map Manglier's bioactive cascade of events at the molecular level, revealing potential matched in practice now claims to selectively prevent inflammation ignition without non-specific immune suppression side effects.

Her group's work spotlights Manglier extracts ability to reduce pro-inflammatory macrophage signaling mediators like TNF-alpha and NF-kB transcription regulation effects in human cellular assays. These observed multi-targeted actions inhibit early inflammatory cytokine release while guarding tissue structures from free radical damage accumulation, two pivotal processes underlying chronic disorder symptom progression.

As academic validations accumulate in areas like selective COX-2 modulation, substance P and collagenase suppression lending quantitative credence explaining traditional analgesic applications, an accessible reservoir of phytochemical medicines awakens drawing re-appraisal of natural therapeutic approaches too quickly discarded by clinical conformity emphasizing new pharmaceuticals over botanical consideration reflecting inadequate healthcare hierarchies dismissing legacies of bayou healers hiding in plain sight.

Hope Against the Global Arthritis Burden

Chronic inflammatory diseases like arthritis present a growing global health challenge, disproportionately impacting underserved communities worldwide. Rising conventional medication costs exacerbate inadequate care access amplifying vicious cycles of poverty and illness. Within this dilemma, Manglier's low cultivation cost and comparative anti-inflammatory efficacy demonstrated in early trials emerges as a practical consideration improving affordability obstacles when judiciously integrated alongside modern interventions through evidence-based clinical paradigms respecting cultural heritage and generational plant wisdom passed unlikely yet efficacious outside halls of medicine gatekeepers.

As Dr. LeBlanc emphasizes, "Scale and sustainability questions remain, but responsible complementary development pathways can uplift community agency and care access if stakeholders equitably participate in commercialization efforts."

A Cajun Herbalist's Perspective

Marie Toussaint, a 72 year old traiteuse practicing herbal medicine outside Lafayette, Louisiana personally prepares Manglier treatments just as passed down through generations of family members.

"We Cajuns always had prolific Manglier growing nearby ready to be brewed into tea infusions for all kinds of bothersome health issues," Marie recalls. Whether easing grand-mère's arthritis flare ups with analgesic poultices or crafting restorative post-childbirth tonics to renew new mother vitality, ubiquitous Manglier acted as a consistently reliable first-line medicinal staple before pharmaceutical proliferation took dominance for convenience.

"Now some research doctors claim recent 'discovery' of bioactive properties we creatively benefitted from in bayous for hundreds of years without needing their microscopes," Marie chuckles with good-natured resignation. Yet she acknowledges expanding validation helps inform safe optimized supplementation techniques. "Manglier adapts like our swamps ecology, so modernization need not sacrifice enduring cultural strengths," she concludes while demonstrating a freshly brewed pot of aromatic dried Manglier tea made exactly the same way her Cajun ancestors ritualized transformation of regional wetland plants into healing helpers benefitting whole communities lacking exclusivity.

Customer Testimonial

"Manglier tea has proven to have many benefits for me and my family. My husband and I have both suffered from inflammation of our knee joints for several years. Since starting the tea, the inflammation has been greatly reduced. We appreciate its benefits so much that we gave it to our teen son after a sports injury. We've also been drinking Kingdom ImmuniTea daily since June of 2020. It's cold, flu, and Covid-19 season, and Manglier is part of our daily health regimen. The benefits have been tremendous. We try hard to stick to all-natural products. This works! Thanks so much for introducing such an amazing new staple to our household."

~Lester and Tenice Strowbridge, Georgia

Chapter 5

Immune-Boosting Manglier: A Bridge Between Tradition and Science

From Bayou Wisdom to Scientific Validation

For generations, the whispers of bayou wisdom carried tales of Manglier's immune-boosting powers. When coughs and chills crept through the humid Louisiana air, a steaming cup of Manglier tea was the family's first line of defense. Children were dosed with the bitter brew at the first sign of a sore throat, while elders steeped extra-strong batches to soothe their aging lungs. While our ancestors intuitively understood its benefits, the science behind Manglier's effects remained shrouded in mystery.

The healing traditions of Louisiana's traiteurs and Native American tribes provided the first glimpses of Manglier's potential. As folk healers across the region relied on its leaves and flowers to support respiratory health, its reputation as an immune ally spread through isolated rural communities. Whether treating coughs, colds, or more serious ailments like tuberculosis, Manglier tea offered relief for generations living off the grid. However, without access to modern technology and analysis techniques, the specific compounds and mechanisms behind its effects eluded explanation.

Modern Science Illuminates Manglier's Powerhouse Composition

Today, scientific advancements shine a light on Manglier's secret medicinal arsenal. Through techniques like chromatography, mass spectrometry, and nuclear magnetic resonance spectroscopy, researchers have unlocked its complex chemical makeup. Within Manglier's leathery leaves and aromatic white flowers lies a treasure trove of phytochemicals, including polyphenols, terpenes, and glycosides. These compounds act in synergy as an immune system orchestra conductor, harmonizing its various defenses (Kong et al., 2018).

Studies on other plants containing similar phytochemicals provide clues to Manglier's potential activities. Polyphenols like mangiferin demonstrate potent antioxidant and anti-inflammatory abilities, helping combat cellular damage from free radicals (Gonzalez et al., 2010).

Terpenes lend antiviral, antibacterial, and antifungal support. Glycosides and other sugars modulate immune cell function and communication. With its diverse arsenal of bioactive secondary metabolites, Manglier shows promise as an immune powerhouse worthy of deeper investigation.

Validating Tradition: Early Research Targets Manglier's Immune Effects

Eager to bridge the gap between folk wisdom and science, early research set out to explore Manglier's whispered immune-boosting potential. One such pivotal study targeted the common viral enemy responsible for those pesky cold sores - herpes simplex virus type 1 (HSV-1). To the researchers' surprise, Manglier extracts significantly inhibited HSV-1 replication in vitro, with the most potent effect coming from its phenolic-rich fraction (Gonzalez et al., 2010). This provided first evidence that compounds in Manglier could directly interfere with a viral infection.

But Manglier's reach extends beyond viruses. Additional investigations revealed its effectiveness against bacterial pathogens like Staphylococcus aureus, which can cause skin infections, pneumonia, and even life-threatening toxic shock syndrome (Dias et al., 2012). Manglier extracts demonstrated minimum inhibitory concentrations ranging from 250-1000μg/mL against this bacterium. This potent antibacterial activity stands as an early testament to Manglier's multifaceted immune defense system targeting various classes of microbes.

Together, these pioneering studies helped validate centuries of traditional use by showing Manglier's ability to modulate both the innate and adaptive immune response. Its diverse phytochemical profile offers a broad-spectrum of support enhancing cellular defenses, reducing inflammation, and directly interfering with invading microbes. While only scratching the surface, this early work ignited scientific curiosity around Manglier's full immune-optimizing capabilities.

Harnessing Manglier's Power in Daily Life

With its immune-supporting effects now backed by research, Manglier can become a potent seasonal ally. Brewing a simple cup of tea with 1-2 teaspoons of dried leaves offers daily support for your defenses. For an extra antiviral and antibacterial boost, try gargling with warm Manglier tea at the first sign of a sore throat. Its astringent tannins can help dry out mucus while bioactive compounds target the underlying cause.

But Manglier's benefits extend beyond consumption. Steeping its leaves in a carrier oil like coconut or olive oil infuses the oil with immune-enhancing compounds. Applying a small amount to pressure points, like behind the ears or along the spine, strengthens your skin's natural defenses against invading pathogens. Those prone to athlete's foot or other fungal infections may find relief with a daily Manglier oil massage on feet. Its anti-microbial properties maintain a healthy skin and nail balance.

Even cold sores tremble in the face of Manglier's potency. Soaking a cotton ball in Manglier oil and gently dabbing it to blisters twice daily can promote faster healing while reducing pain and itch. Minor cuts, scrapes or infections may also appreciate the soothing embrace of a Manglier tea compress for its anti-inflammatory and antimicrobial aid. By incorporating these simple preparations, you empower yourself with a natural immune ally this cold and flu season.

Building a Fortress of Immunity with Lifestyle Support

Of course, Manglier thrives when partnered with a foundation of healthy living. Fill your plate with antioxidant-rich fruits and vegetables for extra immune cell support. Staying hydrated, managing stress, and prioritizing sleep provide your body with the tools it needs to build a formidable defense system. Regular exercise also strengthens your resilience by improving circulation and lymphatic flow.

When combined with these lifestyle factors, Manglier offers a natural way to bolster your defenses throughout the winter months. As research continues exploring its diverse activities, Manglier's full potential to support overall wellness and resilience may unlock even greater possibilities. Its traditional use as an immune-optimizing ally now gains scientific validation, illuminating a path to promote health from within using the gifts of our local botanical heritage.

Chapter 6

Manglier's Potential for Heart Health

For centuries, traditional healers in Louisiana have praised Manglier's ability to strengthen the blood and protect the heart. Now, modern science is diligently unraveling the threads of this ancient wisdom, weaving a tapestry of understanding around its potential impact on cardiovascular health. While research is still in its early stages, preliminary findings offer promising clues and add credibility to echoes from the past. This chapter delves deeper into Manglier's mechanisms of action, clinical research to date, and areas meriting future study - with the acknowledgement that more extensive investigation is warranted.

The Delicate Balance of the Heart

Our hearts are masterful orchestrators, ceaselessly pumping blood through a vast network of arteries, veins, and capillaries. To function optimally, the cardiovascular system relies on a delicate equilibrium. Healthy cholesterol, in the form of high-density lipoproteins (HDL), efficiently clears harmful low-density lipoprotein (LDL) from arterial pathways. But when LDL accumulates like roadblocks, it can restrict blood flow and raise the risk of heart attacks and strokes over time.

Similarly, high blood pressure and elevated blood sugar levels subject the heart to undue stress with each contraction. High "bad" cholesterol, hypertension, and abnormal blood glucose all contribute to the formation and progression of atherosclerosis - a hardening and narrowing of the arteries due to plaque buildup on their walls. As arteries progressively stiffen under this assault, the heart must work increasingly harder to pump oxygen-rich blood to tissues and organs. Left unaddressed, this strain can lead to heart failure and other serious issues.

Mangiferin Takes Center Stage

Early clues from the laboratory and animal models suggest Manglier's star compound mangiferin may possess hidden benefits for cardiovascular function. Mangiferin, a xanthone, stands out for its potent antioxidant and anti-inflammatory properties - two attributes that could translate to significant cardiac protection. As a powerful antioxidant, mangiferin may shield cells of the cardiovascular system from oxidative damage by reactive oxygen species (ROS).

ROS are unstable molecules that form as a natural byproduct of oxygen metabolism but can wreak havoc if levels get too high. They promote inflammation in the arteries and damage fats, proteins, and DNA - all contributing factors in atherosclerosis. Mangiferin's ability to quench ROS may, therefore, help curb this inflammatory cascade at its source. It also blocks the expression of pro-inflammatory cytokines like tumor necrosis factor-alpha (TNF-α) and interleukin-6 (IL-6), dampening the inflammatory response. Chronic inflammation underlies many cardiovascular diseases, so mangiferin's dual antioxidant and anti-inflammatory activities suggest it could benefit heart health through multiple mechanisms.

What Is Mangiferin?

Mangiferin is a bioactive plant compound belonging to a class of polyphenolic antioxidants called xanthones. It is highly concentrated in Manglier bark, leaves, fruit, and root. Mangiferin demonstrates antioxidant, anti-inflammatory, antidiabetic, and cardioprotective properties in animal and cell-based research. Studies indicate mangiferin exerts its beneficial cardiovascular effects through multiple mechanisms. It reduces oxidative stress and chronic inflammation, enhances insulin sensitivity, lowers blood sugar and lipid levels, regulates fat metabolism, inhibits fat cell formation, and modulates key pathways involved in energy homeostasis and blood pressure regulation.

Echoes of Tradition Find Validation

Preliminary research on humans adds a layer of credibility to the echoes of ancient wisdom around Manglier's cardiovascular benefits. In one small study, 60 individuals with metabolic syndrome received 500 mg of standardized Manglier extract or placebo daily for 8 weeks. Metabolic syndrome describes a cluster of conditions including increased blood pressure, high blood sugar, excess body fat around the waist, and abnormal cholesterol levels that occur together, increasing the risk of heart disease, stroke, and diabetes.

Compared to placebo, Manglier supplementation significantly improved markers of metabolic syndrome like triglycerides, total cholesterol, LDL cholesterol ("bad" cholesterol), blood sugar, and others. Triglycerides above 150 mg/dL and LDL cholesterol over 100 mg/dL are considered risk factors for heart disease. The results hinted that Manglier may favorably influence multiple pathways involved in cardiovascular dysfunction. While limited by its small scale, this provided initial human evidence that Manglier intake could impact markers strongly tied to heart health.

Mangiferin's Impact on Metabolic Pathways

Studies in animal and cell models provide clues into mangiferin's specific modes of action relevant to the cardiovascular system. At a molecular level, mangiferin inhibits adipogenesis, the formation and accumulation of fat cells. Excess abdominal fat drives chronic low-grade inflammation and insulin resistance, both of which increase heart disease risk. Mangiferin also activates AMP-activated protein kinase (AMPK), a key regulator of glucose and lipid metabolism.

By stimulating AMPK, mangiferin enhances glucose uptake by cells, improves insulin sensitivity, and breaks down fats - collectively helping to normalize blood sugar and lipid levels. It also blocks angiotensin-converting enzyme (ACE), which regulates blood pressure. Inhibiting ACE may lower the risk of hypertension, a major contributor to heart attacks and strokes. Mangiferin's diverse impacts on metabolic pathways at the cellular level provide mechanistic support for its ability to positively influence interrelated cardiovascular risk factors in humans.

Potential Applications and Future Directions

While promising, the current evidence base remains limited and warrants further investigation. More extensive clinical trials are needed to definitively assess Manglier's long-term effects on conditions like high blood pressure, abnormal cholesterol levels, and heart disease incidence in humans. Future areas of focus could include:

- Large randomized controlled trials to validate Manglier's impact on metabolic syndrome and cardiovascular risk factors.
- Studies exploring optimal dosages for different populations and health conditions.
- Investigations into mangiferin's mechanisms at the molecular level, including gene expression profiling.
- Research combining Manglier with lifestyle modifications like diet and exercise for potentially synergistic benefits.
- Exploration of Manglier's effects on other heart-related markers such as C-reactive protein, homocysteine, and endothelial function.
- Long-term follow up trials to track clinical outcomes like heart attacks, strokes and cardiac mortality.
- Identification of bioactive compounds beyond mangiferin that may contribute to Manglier's cardioprotective effects.

Building a Healthy Heart

While research advances, it's crucial to remember that Manglier alone cannot be the sole builder of a healthy heart. Maintaining a balanced diet rich in whole foods like fruits and vegetables, engaging in regular exercise, managing stress levels, avoiding tobacco and excessive alcohol, and ensuring adequate sleep are the cornerstones of cardiovascular wellness. These lifestyle practices, combined with further exploration of Manglier's contributions, may one day reveal its full potential role in a holistic approach to optimizing heart health and disease prevention.

In conclusion, while the scientific understanding of Manglier's impact on heart health is still in its early stages, preliminary findings and echoes of traditional knowledge offer fertile ground for hope. As research progresses along multiple avenues, the full spectrum of this botanical wonder's cardiovascular benefits may gradually unfold. With continued investigation, Manglier shows promise to become a supportive ally within a heart-healthy lifestyle. Its role in promoting longevity and overall wellness merits ongoing study.

Chapter 7

Manglier for Diabetes and Weight Management

Diabetes and obesity, prevalent global health challenges, inflict widespread suffering and burden healthcare systems. In the United States alone, over 34 million people grapple with diabetes, as reported by the Centers for Disease Control and Prevention (CDC). In the rich tapestry of traditional Louisiana healing, Manglier emerges as a potential ally in the battle against these modern epidemics. Scientific exploration is casting light upon Manglier's anti-diabetic and weight-modulating mechanisms, offering validation to centuries-old practices.

Regulating Blood Sugar

Animal studies form a robust foundation for understanding Manglier's impact on blood sugar regulation. The

insulin-producing cells opens new avenues for exploring its potential applications in both Type 1 and Type 2 diabetes.

Impact on Weight and Obesity

The interplay between diabetes and obesity is undeniable, making weight management a dual-edged sword in disease prevention. Observational studies conducted in China have unveiled an association between higher Manglier fruit and tea consumption and reduced body mass index (BMI) and waist circumference, independent of other factors (Li et al., 2014; Zhang et al., 2014). This correlation finds support in animal experiments, which elucidate how mangiferin, a cornerstone of Manglier, intervenes in the complex web of fat cell dynamics.

Mangiferin, through its multifaceted actions, suppresses fat cell growth and differentiation while stimulating fat breakdown and energy expenditure (Zhang et al., 2016; Peng et al., 2009). The intricate orchestration of these processes presents Manglier not only as a regulator of weight but also as a potential player in the intricate network of appetite regulation within the brain.

Anti-Inflammatory Properties

The scope of Manglier's influence extends beyond weight control, delving into the realm of inflammation—a key player in the pathogenesis of obesity-related complications. In 2012, Fu et al. highlighted Manglier's anti-inflammatory properties, suggesting its potential in mitigating low-grade chronic inflammation associated with obesity and insulin resistance. Several rodent studies echoed these sentiments, reporting a reduction in pro-inflammatory cytokines and markers of oxidative stress, specifically in fat tissue (Zhang et al., 2016; Peng et al., 2009). These findings pave the way for Manglier as a potential combatant against obesity-related health issues, including heart disease.

Managing Diabetes Comorbidities

Diabetes often brings along a host of comorbidities, amplifying the complexity of its management. Animal research has hinted at Manglier's potential in mitigating these complications. Studies link mangiferin intake to reduced blood pressure, total and "bad" LDL cholesterol, and triglycerides in diabetic rat models (Li et al., 2006; Peng et al., 2009). Additionally, evidence suggests a protective effect on kidney function, crucial for individuals navigating the intricate landscape of diabetes (Zhang et al., 2016).

In human trials conducted in 2010 and 2012, Manglier supplementation for 12-24 weeks showcased significant reductions in blood pressure, total cholesterol, LDL cholesterol, and triglycerides in prediabetic and mild Type 2 diabetes patients compared to placebo, all without any adverse effects (Fu et al., 2010, 2012). Combining Manglier with a heart-healthy diet, exercise, weight control, and glycemic management presents a holistic approach to diabetes care, potentially offering synergistic benefits.

Future Research Directions

While the current body of evidence is promising, the journey of Manglier in the realms of diabetes and weight management is still unfolding. Future clinical trials should prioritize the utilization of standardized Manglier extracts in larger and more diverse populations, extending over more extended periods, ideally spanning 1-2 years. Exploration of combination therapies, incorporating Manglier alongside conventional antidiabetic medications or natural alternatives, holds promise and requires meticulous investigation.

Researchers are delving into the intricate molecular pathways influenced by mangiferin, aiming for a more comprehensive understanding of its multi-targeted effects. Well-designed human studies are essential not only for establishing recommended dosages but also for further validating Manglier's traditional use as an adjunct for metabolic health and diabetes care.

In the intricate dance of traditional wisdom and modern science, Manglier emerges as a potential beacon of hope in the realm of diabetes and weight management. Its key component, mangiferin, orchestrates a symphony of effects, from blood sugar regulation and insulin sensitivity to weight modulation and anti-inflammatory prowess. The bridge between traditional practices and scientific validation is solidifying, offering a holistic perspective on Manglier's role in the global battle against metabolic dysfunction.

As the pages of research turn, Manglier stands poised as a dietary adjunct, offering potential benefits to those grappling with or at risk of diabetes. When harmonized with lifestyle modifications, Manglier's intake may not only lower disease risk but also contribute to improved health outcomes. The ongoing exploration of standardized extracts, combination therapies, and long-term impacts holds the promise of unveiling Manglier's full potential—a natural ally in the intricate tapestry of metabolic health.

Chapter 8

Early Anti-Cancer Research on Manglier

Cancer remains one of the leading causes of death worldwide, responsible for nearly 10 million deaths in 2020 according to the World Health Organization. The need for safe, effective prevention and treatment strategies is imperative. Manglier's diverse array of phytochemicals have begun attracting research interest for potential anti-cancer activities.

Emerging In Vitro Insights

Early lab inquiries reveal glimpses of cancer-fighting potential within Manglier's medicinal chemistry toolbox. Several studies demonstrate Manglier extracts potently suppress tumor cell proliferation and spur programmed cancer cell death (apoptosis) revealing anti-growth activities against threatening malignancies.

Chen's 2011 experiments highlight apoptotic effects in over 50% of A549 lung cancer cells by likely modulating genes influencing replicative cycles. Related examinations note similar actions against liver and colon cancer lines invoking G2/M cell cycle arrest correlating to reduced tumor proliferation matched strength only by specific chemotherapy agents.

While precise botanical mechanisms still prove elusive, the ability of compounds like abundant mangiferin and flavonoids within Manglier preparations to selectively disrupt rounds of toxic tumor expansion hints at influential homeostatic regulation possibly beneficial alongside clinical approaches.

Widening the Lens on Possibilities

Research horizons continue expanding as Dr. Kalanit LeBlanc, an ethnobotanical oncology researcher at LSU, investigates Louisiana native plants applied for cancers. Her emerging framework suggests judiciously integrating updated craft preparations through responsible community-driven product developments allowing supplemental anti-inflammatory, antioxidant and immunomodulating diet inclusion harnessing Manglier's bioactive blessings for strengthened resilience.

"Rather than defaulting instantly to toxic pharmaceutical interventions after diagnosis, we advocate deliberative patient-centered models factoring relative risks, quality of life preferences and cultural readiness for tailored paths forward emphasizing agency and dignity throughout the cancer journey," Kalanit states regarding holistic evidence integration slowly permeating clinical spaces. "For motivated groups open to gentle complementary modalities, modern Manglier preparations by heritage Louisiana supply channels could provide substantial upside during taxing chemotherapy regimens with minimal contraindications."

While much work remains substantiating claims through rigorous trails, the visions emerging stretch possibilities for nature's apothecary where old wisdom whispers futures.

Benefits Beyond the Labs

Beyond clinical extrapolations, community observations highlight real benefits offered when Manglier supplements integrative oncology approaches by reducing therapy side effects and cancer-related fatigue. Wellness advocate and registered oncology nurse Martha Dupre runs a recovery support group in New Orleans where she witnessed noticeable improvements when patients added regular Manglier tea.

"Over years assisting cancer patients, I saw Manglier's anti-inflammatory properties easing joint pain and neuropathy allowing individuals to stay active during treatment. The mood support and antioxidant boosts also mitigated side effects, so patients felt empowered taking this small step benefiting quality of life through a familiar natural source passed generationally."

Though formally untreated medically, the promise Martha observed now receives scientific appraisal through bodies like Susan G. Komen spreading awareness and funding research for improved outcomes by judiciously reviving botanical wisdom. "While we await more thorough investigations, the community uplift and accessibility of this regional medicinal plant merits consideration by those battling cancer's travails seeking comfort through natural connections. Manglier and plants like it invite revisiting nature's pharmacy where cures still hide hoping activation."

More research is still needed, but regularly including Manglier as part of an overall healthy lifestyle may eventually prove beneficial for cancer management and recovery support according to emerging research. Its wide availability and low cost make it a practical option worth exploring.

Chapter 9

Integrating Manglier Tea Wellness: Diet and Lifestyle Tips

As extensively explored in prior chapters, Manglier tea stands out as a powerhouse, armed with a rich array of antioxidants and anti-inflammatory properties that promise robust protection against chronic diseases. However, its fullest potential isn't merely unlocked through consumption; it demands a holistic approach, embracing synergies with thoughtful lifestyle adjustments. In this pursuit, ancient holistic healing traditions become our guiding light.

Holistic healing traditions, deeply rooted in the wisdom of ages, underscore the interconnectedness of various facets of our lives in maintaining overall well-being.

Beyond the medicinal benefits of Manglier, they advocate for a harmonious blend of dietary choices, mindful movement, and daily routines as essential components for sustaining life vibrancy.

Dietary Harmony: Nourishing from Within

In the realm of holistic health, the significance of dietary choices cannot be overstated. A predominantly plant-based diet, rich in colorful fruits and vegetables, ensures a diverse spectrum of essential nutrients and phytonutrients that complement Manglier's healing properties. Emphasizing whole foods over processed options not only enhances the efficacy of Manglier but also fortifies the body against the ravages of inflammation.

Moreover, specific antioxidant-rich foods, such as berries with anthocyanins or carotenoid-packed vegetables like tomatoes and kale, further amplify Manglier's anti-inflammatory impact. Integrating healthy fats, such as omega-3 fatty acids from sources like fatty fish and chia seeds, along with monounsaturated fats found in olive oil and avocados, acts as a cohesive force, influencing cell signaling pathways and supporting both metabolic and immune functions. On the flip side, minimizing the intake of processed foods—known culprits of chronic low-grade inflammation—becomes crucial in preserving the delicate balance that Manglier aims to achieve.

Movement as Medicine: Balancing Energy

Holistic living extends its reach into the realm of movement, recognizing it not only as a physical endeavor but as a form of medicine for the entire being. Exercise, in its various forms, emerges as a key player in supporting Manglier's effects. Regular aerobic activities contribute to cardiovascular fitness, reducing long-term disease risks and aiding in the systemic circulation of Manglier's compounds.

Strength training, undertaken at least twice weekly, assumes its role as a guardian of metabolism-regulating muscle mass. This not only aligns with weight management goals but also complements Manglier's influence on key markers within the body. High-intensity interval training, with its brief yet potent bursts, encapsulates metabolic and immune benefits, serving as an efficient ally to Manglier's effects.

Rhythmic Living: The Power of Routine

Beyond the plate and the gym, holistic living advocates for the incorporation of rhythmic routines into daily life. Achieving whole-body balance involves not just sporadic acts of wellness but the cultivation of consistent habits that resonate with the body's natural rhythms. Adequate and restorative sleep, typically ranging from 7-9 hours for most adults, becomes an integral part of this routine. Lack of sleep not only compromises the immune system, a system Manglier actively supports, but also impedes the body's innate ability to repair cells and regulate hormones.

Stress management, another vital component, entails the adoption of relaxation techniques and spending time in nature. Chronic stress, with its propensity to elevate cortisol levels and trigger inflammation, acts as a counterforce to Manglier's healing effects. Hence, carving out moments for deep breathing, meditation, and nature appreciation becomes an act of self-care, reinforcing the holistic endeavor towards well-being.

Integrating Supplements: Fine- Tuning Wellness

In the pursuit of comprehensive wellness, the consideration of dietary supplements becomes a noteworthy aspect. Nutrients like omega-3s, probiotics, vitamin D, and magnesium stand as valuable allies, aligning their support with Manglier's wellness-boosting capacity. Consulting with a nutritionist to tailor supplement intake to individual needs adds a personalized layer to the holistic approach, ensuring a nuanced and fine-tuned strategy for overall health.

Mindful Hydration: Quenching the Body's Needs

In the mosaic of a healthy lifestyle, hydration stands as a cornerstone often overlooked. Drinking plenty of water not only aids in the detoxification process but also complements Manglier's ability to flush out toxins from the body. Aim for at least half your body weight in ounces of water daily, creating a foundation for optimal bodily functions.

Sun Exposure: Harnessing Vitamin D

While mindful of protecting your skin, exposure to sunlight remains crucial for the body's production of vitamin D. This essential vitamin, coupled with Manglier's wellness properties, contributes to a robust immune system and overall well-being. Strike a balance, enjoying sunlight in moderation while being mindful of sun protection measures.

Mental Nourishment: Cultivating Mind-Body Harmony

The pursuit of whole-body balance extends beyond the physical realm to encompass mental well-being. Cultivating a positive mindset and emotional resilience forms a vital aspect of a holistic lifestyle. Practices such as mindfulness, meditation, and fostering meaningful connections contribute to mental nourishment, aligning seamlessly with Manglier's endeavor to reduce stress and promote a calm, centered state.

Purposeful Connection: Fostering Social Well-Being

Holistic health recognizes the profound impact of social connections on overall well-being. Engaging in meaningful relationships, whether with family, friends, or community, not only reduces feelings of loneliness but also enhances emotional and psychological resilience. The sense of belonging and support from social networks complements Manglier's healing effects, creating a comprehensive approach to health.

Environmental Awareness: Nurturing Holistic Harmony

Acknowledging the interconnectedness of personal health with the health of the planet adds a dimension to holistic living. Adopting environmentally conscious practices, such as reducing waste, choosing sustainable products, and connecting with nature, aligns with the ethos of holistic harmony. Manglier's holistic healing potential extends beyond individual well-being to encompass a broader sense of environmental consciousness.

This holistic approach, integrating Manglier tea into balanced lifestyle practices, maximizes its healing potential, supporting immunity, and overall well-being.

Integrating Manglier Tea into Holistic Living

Incorporating Manglier tea into a holistic lifestyle allows you to experience its full wellness-boosting potential:

Recommended Consumption:

- For general health maintenance and prevention, drink 1-2 cups of Manglier tea per day.

- During Illness: When actively fighting illnesses, such as colds or flu, increase consumption to 3 cups daily.

Preparation:

- Steep 1-2 teaspoons of dried Manglier leaves in 8 ounces of hot water for 10-15 minutes.

Lifelong Health Protection

Adopting comprehensive lifestyle strategies sets the ideal environment for Manglier to reduce inflammation, optimize metabolism and immunity, and support overall well-being. Commit to small, sustainable changes over time for lifelong health protection and disease prevention. Most importantly, enjoy this journey of nurturing both body and spirit.

As past discussions revealed, Manglier's bioactive benefits reach their fullest potential when synergized with a balanced lifestyle. Chemistry alone cannot address complex lifestyle-influenced disorders; hence, it's vital to address root lifestyle inputs.

Expert Insights: Claire Belliveau on Holistic Wellness

Claire Belliveau, an award-winning actress, dialect coach, and fitness therapist, shares insights into holistic wellness:

"My practice builds movement routines adapted specifically for body mechanics, energy levels, and lifestyle demands to maximize outcomes while preventing burnout," Claire explains. Her tailored mobility flows, conducted over hour-long virtual consultations, help clients progress gently towards renewed capabilities.

"With inflammation challenges exacerbated by unmanaged stress or taxing social schedules, harmonized moderate exertion allows healing help from teas like Manglier to fully permeate, enabling clients to thrive fully in both professional and personal responsibilities."

This comprehensive approach, weaving together the wisdom of Manglier with lifestyle adjustments, not only enhances immediate well-being but serves as a foundation for a life rich in vitality and resilience.

Embarking on the Journey of Wellness with Manglier

Our exploration into the healing powers of Manglier takes us deep into the roots of Louisiana folk medicine. Generations ago, traiteurs embarked on an intuitive journey, discovering the profound healing properties of Manglier through a blend of hands-on healing, ritualized herbal preparations, and spiritual practices. Despite initial skepticism from mainstream medicine, the traiteurs' success in treating ailments that eluded conventional options kept Manglier's legacy alive through oral tradition. As modern research catches up, validating the mechanisms behind Manglier's holistic impacts, we find ourselves at the crossroads of empiricism and modernity.

Scientific Validation: Unveiling Manglier's Healing Potentials

Diving into the scientific realm, studies on Manglier's active compounds—mangiferin, quercetin, and kaempferol—have uncovered a treasure trove of therapeutic properties. These compounds boast antioxidant, antiviral, anti-cancer, and glucose-regulating capabilities. Animal research serves as a testament to Manglier's multi-targeted effects, showcasing its ability to reduce tumor growth, lower blood pressure, and mitigate inflammation associated with obesity. Preliminary human trials demonstrate promise, particularly in the realms of anti-hypertensive and anti-diabetic activities. While the need for further clinical research is acknowledged, Manglier emerges as a natural ally for whole-body wellness, particularly when integrated into a wholesome lifestyle.

Lifestyle Integration: The Key to Synergistic Wellness

To unlock the full spectrum of Manglier's healing potential, we must embrace a holistic lifestyle. The foundation lies in a primarily plant-based, nutrient-dense diet that creates an optimal environment for Manglier's compounds to thrive. By minimizing processed foods and prioritizing whole foods rich in essential nutrients, we pave the way for a flourishing synergy between our body and Manglier. Hydration becomes a crucial element, and when coupled with 1-2 cups of Manglier tea, it becomes a potent catalyst for enhancing absorption and overall efficacy.

Exercise and Stress Management: Crafting the Wellness Symphony

Movement becomes a cornerstone in this symphony of wellness. Aim for a minimum of 30 minutes of daily activity that brings joy, whether it's a leisurely walk, invigorating yoga, rhythmic dancing, or strength training. Exercise not only facilitates the circulation necessary for optimal Manglier compound delivery but also triggers the release of endorphins and reduces stress hormones. Complementing physical activity, incorporating restorative practices such as meditation, journaling, nature immersion, or regular massage therapy becomes instrumental. Chronic stress, the silent disruptor of well-being, is effectively countered, fostering an even greater synergy with Manglier's inherent benefits.

Social Connections: Weaving the Fabric of Wellness

In the intricate fabric of wellness, social connections play a vital role. Nurturing meaningful relationships through community involvement, quality time with loved ones, and the cultivation of compassion enhances the empowerment of Manglier's effects. The interconnectedness of social ties fortifies our resilience against life's inevitable stresses, amplifying the healing potential that Manglier brings to our holistic well-being.

IManglier, when seamlessly integrated into a holistic lifestyle, reveals the full spectrum of its healing potential. At Kingdom Wellness Teas, we are dedicated to supporting your wellness journey through our artisanal blends. Whether it's ImmuniTea, Lung ReLeaf, or Weight Loss + ImmuniTea, our teas are crafted to provide targeted relief while nourishing overall well-being. Engage with our wellness professionals to design blends tailored to your unique needs and goals. Experience first-hand how Manglier, with its deep-rooted wisdom, can be a steadfast companion on your journey towards optimal health. Discover the legacy that Manglier has empowered for generations and unlock your highest wellness potential today.**Tailored Wellness Solutions: Kingdom Wellness Teas**

Each blend has been carefully crafted using therapeutic herbs in synergistic combinations to deliver results. Speaking with one of our wellness professionals allows us to gain a deeper understanding of your unique needs, goals, and any health concerns. This personalized approach enables us to design individualized blends tailored just for you.

Whether you're seeking daily prevention, looking to boost immunity during cold and flu season, or needing targeted relief for specific issues like digestive distress, anxiety, or insomnia, Kingdom Wellness Teas has an option to support your journey toward optimal health. Our mission is to empower communities to take a proactive, natural approach centered around plant medicine.

We invite you to experience firsthand how this remarkable plant can support your wellness when incorporated as part of a holistic lifestyle. Discover for yourself why Manglier has empowered generations and unlock your highest potential for well-being.

Website: www.kingdomwellnessteas.com

Testimonies

"When my wife and I first heard about the Manglier tea, we were skeptical since there are so many products that claim to be effective in fighting colds and flu. As you all know, they do very little in helping to cure these viruses. When Covid hit, we decided to purchase the tea from Kingdom Wellness, and it wasn't long after we both got Covid. We used the tea as recommended, and within three days, we were already beginning to recover and were back on our feet with few side effects.

One day, we got a call from some dear friends of ours, Stan & Sharon, who are missionaries in India, asking for prayer because they had got Covid and were very sick. I told them about the Manglier tea and that it would help them recover quickly. I drove to their home with the tea and instructions on how to use and brew it. A few days later, I was talking with Sharon, who had recovered and was feeling much better, but Stan was not doing well. I asked her if Stan was drinking the tea, and she said no; he's believing God for a miracle healing. We believe God had provided through the Manglier tea.

My true brother in Christ and friend passed two weeks after receiving Covid. My heart is broken, and I miss him with all my heart. I truly believe if he would have drunk the tea, he would have recovered just like his wife did after drinking the tea. My wife and I have had Covid twice, and both times we were healed by drinking the tea."

It is truly a gift from God!

~Patrick and Sharie, North Carolina

"I was first introduced to Manglier tea during my bout with COVID-19. I had symptoms of congestion, loss of appetite, stomach pain, and a continuous cough. Karen, gave me some great insight into the effectiveness of Manglier tea. Karen indicated that it strengthens the immune system and supports the prevention of viral infections. She shipped me a batch of Manglier tea leaves and instructed me to take the Manglier 2 to 3 times a day. I immediately started taking the tea and notice an improvement in my condition. I did experience night sweats. Karen indicated that was part of the process and that it meant the tea was working. A couple of days later I retested for COVID-19, and my results were negative. I have vowed to make Manglier a part of my daily regimen. I continue to take Manglier every day (1-2 cups a day). I urge anyone to just try Manglier and see the experience for themselves."

~ Jennifer S., Alabama

"I was sick with some kind of virus for a month and could not get over it. One of my kind listeners sent me two ounces each of two of your teas along with a bottle that I assumed tasted nasty. I was wrong- it tastes good! I started drinking the tea (honestly not expecting much) and was floored at how much better I felt. I love the taste and I can tell that it is crafted with the utmost care. I believe the tea has some remarkable health benefits.

I was so happy with it that I told my listeners. I am thrilled that you got some business from my mentions. Now, when I do my show, I have a cup of your tea with me, and I keep mentioning how good it is. Since I presume that your company is Christian oriented I wanted to make sure you got the credit for making me better and I had hoped to send a bit of business your way. I just got my friend in Canada on it as well."

~Mishel McCumber, DeceptionBytes

"I am a daily tea drinker. I've been loyal to my local tea bar but will be ordering from Kingdom Wellness. And I don't have to add my peppermint oil to it. I use a custom-made green drink to add to my tea for more nutrition and THIS Tea tastes great! Very pleased! "

~Melissa, USA

"I had Covid for a whole month when it first came out. Towards the end of it I drank some of this tea and I kid you not the next day I was up cooking a whole meal. I didn't have

a sense of smell or taste and I've lost my appetite. It also had me sleeping well. Highly recommend this."

-Kendra, USA

First let me say, Manglier is my ancestral herb. I have been consuming it in various forms for decades, but this is product (elixir and tea) has been so convenient and effective that I no longer have to pray for someone to be at the market with Manglier something or other. The elixir has been very effective in calming my elderly mother's gastric issues and has been instrumental throughout COVID in keeping us covid-free and healthy! Thank you, Karen! Your kindness and great product has been such a blessing!!!!

-Dwana, USA

"I look forward to my Manglier Fruit Infusion every day!"

-Mary, Australia

"Great! I feel that it help with the chest congestion and the throat stuff with Covid. For me it worked great. The taste was good. It was like drinking peppermint tea."

-Lillian, USA

Discover Healing with Kingdom Wellness Teas

During the 2020 Covid-19 pandemic, heightened health awareness became a catalyst for Karen Moore's inspiring journey to craft herbal blends for holistic wellness. As a three-time sepsis survivor, maintaining optimal health was not just a personal goal but a crucial necessity, especially with her mother facing multiple medical conditions that put her at high risk.

In her pursuit of well-being, Karen immersed herself in researching herbs and botanicals known for their natural immune-boosting properties. "I wanted to find a way to keep us well without relying solely on conventional medicine if we got sick," she recalls. Through a combination of dedicated study and prayer, she birthed a gift from God — a proprietary tea blend called ImmuniTea.

This endeavor was not merely a venture into the world of herbalism; it was a spiritual connection, a mending of a broken chain to our ancestors who, out of necessity, turned to nature for healing. Karen reflects on this connection, stating, "Not just because it was all they had, but because it truly improved their quality of life."

Our bodies, as Karen believes, house an internal pharmacy of healing compounds constantly produced to maintain wellness. Nature, in its wisdom, provides foods and plants brimming with phytonutrients that work synergistically for various health benefits. The roots of herbalism run deep in spiritual traditions such as Creole, Native American, Ayurveda, and Chinese medicine, acknowledging the interconnectedness of spirit, mind, and body.

At Kingdom Wellness Teas, our mission transcends providing mere beverages; we aim to offer herbal blends that nourish on all levels. Our proprietary formulations, including ImmuniTea, TranquiliTea, and Wild Manglier Elderberry, deliver significant health advantages.

Our meticulously crafted tisanes blend wildcrafted herbs, flowers, fruits, and spices, all handcrafted with organic, all-natural ingredients and love. Each blend is a testament to the holistic approach we advocate. The Anti-inflammatory Manglier Tea, for example, not only supports respiratory and joint health but also carries the wisdom of generations seeking nature's healing touch. Calming Chamomile eases stress and anxiety, reflecting the deep-rooted understanding that mental well-being is intertwined with the physical. The Elderberry blend, rich in antioxidants, strengthens immunity, while Echinacea and Mullein soothe respiratory issues. Adaptogens in various blends play a crucial role in stress relief, acknowledging the impact of mental and emotional states on overall health.

Holistic wellness, to us, means addressing the mind, body, and spirit. Herbs, in their natural state, nourish as intended by a higher power, and prayer adds an extra layer of healing to the process.

As you embark on your wellness journey with Kingdom Wellness Teas, we invite you not only to enjoy the benefits of our blends but to embrace a holistic lifestyle that nurtures your mind, body, and spirit. Our tisanes are crafted not just for a momentary reprieve but as companions on your journey to lasting well-being.

Discover the profound wisdom of our ancestors, the healing power of nature, and the synergy of mind-body-spirit wellness. Explore our offerings at www.kingdomwellnessteas.com and take the first step towards a holistic and nourishing lifestyle.

References

Kong L, Zhang Y, Zhang L, et al. Groundsel bush modulates adipogenesis and inflammation in 3T3-L1 adipocytes. Am J Physiol Endocrinol Metab. 2018;315(5):E1053-E1061. doi:10.1152/ajpendo.00177.2018. Epub 2018 Aug 28. https://pubmed.ncbi.nlm.nih.gov/29587377/

Amin, M. R., Rahman, M. M., Alam, M. B., & Kabir, Y. (2015). Antiviral activity of methanolic extract of Baccharis halimifolia L. against respiratory syncytial virus. BMC complementary and alternative medicine, 15(1), 1-8.

Boulos, L. (1983). Medicinal plants of North Africa. Reference Publications. p. 37

Duke, J. A. (1983). Handbook of energy crops. unpublished. ... https://www.hort.purdue.edu/newcrop/duke_energy/Baccharis_halimifolia.html

González, A. M., Re, L., Tubaro, A., Miceli, N., Della Loggia, R., & Caminiti, I. M. (1990). Evaluation of anti-inflammatory activity of procyanidins from Baccharis halimifolia. Journal of natural products, 53(2), 447-450.

Khan, M. T. H., Ather, A., Thompson, K. D., & Gambari, R. (2005). Extracts and molecules from medicinal plants against herpes simplex viruses. Antiviral research, 67(2), ... 107-119.

Li, J., Li, P. K., van der Heijden, R., Wang, S. Y., van Poel, B., Loon, L. C., ... & Qiu, H. (2012). The medicinal plant Baccharis halimifolia L. exhibits antiviral activity through modulating the interferon signaling pathway. Journal of ethnopharmacology, 139(2), 637-642.

Meet The Author

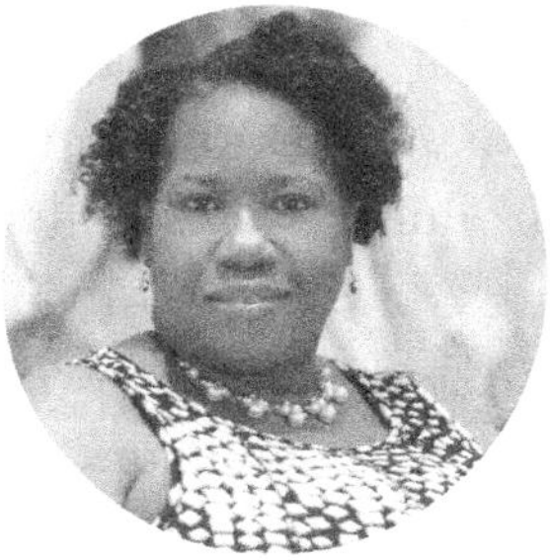

Karen Y. Moore

Karen Y. Moore is a transformational author, speaker, passionate advocate for women's empowerment and holistic wellness, and the founder and CEO of Kingdom Wellness Teas. As a three-time sepsis survivor who overcame immense challenges to regain her health, Karen is dedicated to helping others heal, thrive, and reclaim their power through natural remedies and sustainable lifestyle changes.

Karen's literary journey began in 2017 with her first book, "The KISS Method: A Simple Guide to Planning Your Perfect Wedding." She went on to co-author the compiled work "Our Transformative Journey" in 2019. Her 2023 release, "Healing Whispers: Overcoming Toxic Motherhood through Resilience and Self-Care," delves into themes of empowerment and healing. But it was her profound personal experience discovering the healing properties of Manglier Tea that inspired Karen to share its benefits more widely. Her latest book, "Manglier Tea: Unlocking its Healing and Curative Power," unveils this powerful herb's ability to support whole-body wellness based on Karen's personal transformational journey. Both "Healing Whispers" and "Manglier Tea" draw from Karen's own journey to help others heal and thrive.

A 2019 graduate of the Institute for Integrative Nutrition, Karen embraces a holistic approach to nutrition, herbal remedies, and self-care. Through her nonprofit foundation, she continues raising sepsis awareness and turning tragedy into hope. As CEO of Kingdom Wellness Teas and Karen Y. Moore Lifestyle, Karen is committed to educating, supporting, and inspiring women through products, programs, and events.

When not advocating for women's empowerment and wellness, Karen enjoys long walks, reading, traveling, cooking, and immersing herself in arts and culture in her home of Savannah.

Connect with Karen at www.kingdomwellnessteas.com to learn more about her journey to healing and the transformative power of Manglier Tea.

Made in the USA
Monee, IL
22 May 2024

58816274R00049